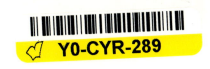

AFRICAN ELEPHANTS

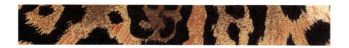

Written by Eduard Zingg

Published by Abdo & Daughters, 6535 Cecilia Circle, Edina, Minnesota 55439

Copyright © 1993 by World Wild Life Films (Pty.) Limited, Postfach 6586, 8023 Zurich, Switzerland

Edited By: Jim Abdo and Bob Italia for Abdo & Daughters Publishing

Text and Photographs: Eduard Zingg
Illustrations and Maps: W. Michel and K. Wozniak

Library of Congress Cataloging-in-Publication Data

Zingg, Eduard, 1940-
    African elephants / written by Eduard Zingg: edited by Bob Italia.
        p.   cm. -- (An African animal adventure)
    Includes index.
    Summary: The author recounts his experiences on expeditions in Botswana and describes some of the animals found there.
    ISBN 1-56239-216-6
    1. African elephant -- Botswana -- Juvenile literature. 2. Mammals-- Botswana -- Juvenile literature. [1. Zoology -- Botswana.
2. Botswana -- Description and travel.]   I. Italia, Robert, 1955-
II. Title.   III. Series: Zingg, Eduard, 1940-   African animal adventure.
QL737.P98Z56 1993
599.6'1 -- dc20   93-3699
                                                       CIP
                                                        AC

Table of Contents

I once saw a female leopard walking along the edge of a river. Her tail was raised in a graceful loop to expose the white underside. It was as if she was holding a torch up high to light the way for her cubs which were following.

THE FEMALE AFRICAN LEOPARD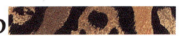

The female African leopard usually produces one to six cubs which are born blind with short tails. After about three months the cubs begin to hunt small animals like frogs and grasshoppers. Cubs are fed on meat mixed with hair and feathers, regurgitated for them by their mother. By the time the cubs are five months old, their mother has taught them how to kill medium-sized prey. Before they are one year old, they are taking part in active hunting. Leopards become independent from about twenty months old, when they spend more time on their own. But they still hunt in the same area.

Leopards develop faster than lions. The cubs take part in hunting at an earlier age. Many young leopards are driven from their group at a young age. They must wander until they find an area of their own in which to hunt. This social structure applies to most meat eaters.

Leopards will make a wide range of kills, including other meat eaters. Lions will kill and eat leopard cubs, and also one another. When leopard males fight over a territory, one may be killed and eaten by the other. When leopard cubs die they may be eaten by the mother.

The leopard relies more on vision and hearing than smell. Hearing is its most important sense in finding its prey. The leopard travels at a walking pace of about 3 miles/hr. (4.8 kilometers/hr.). Sometimes it breaks into a trot, but it seldom keeps this up for long.

The leopard is a creature of careful habits, changing its hunting areas to a fixed plan. This allows the animals in the original hunting area to settle down before it strikes again. Leopards avoid humans wherever possible. If people are in the area they will lie very still in a tree until they go by. But if it is spotted, it is inclined to attack. It is impossible to frighten a leopard away with a shot in the air. It must be killed. Leopards attack with full force, using all four paws and its jaws. Man-eating leopards have seldom been heard of in southern Africa.

You won't find leopards when lions are around. Leopards remain undercover to escape the lions. These two cats greatly dislike each other.

With its cat-like walk, the leopard is the most powerful, aggressive and courageous of all African animals. It is also one of the most beautiful. Its beauty is its biggest disadvantage. Its skin gets a very high price, and has for many centuries. Despite its intelligence, the leopard is fairly easily caught in a trap.

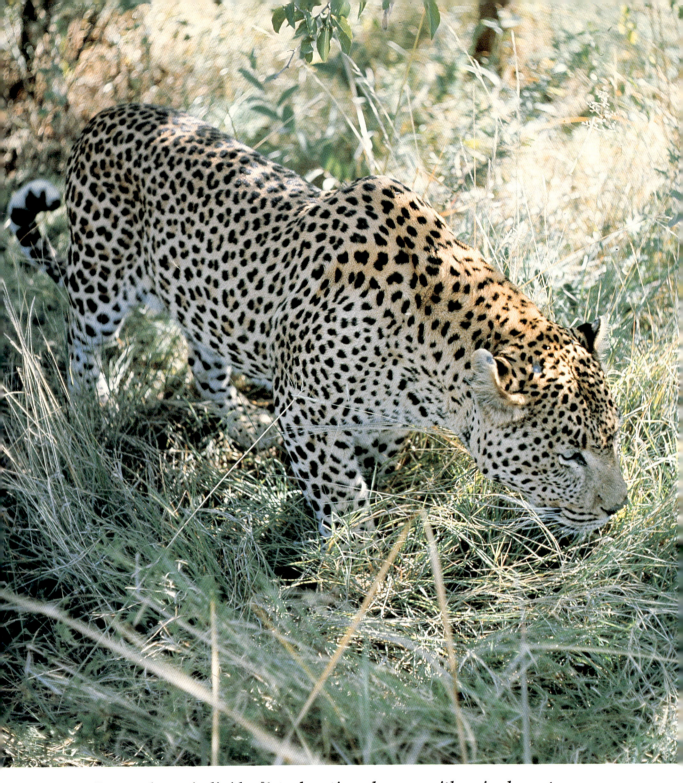

Leopards are individualists, hunting alone or with a single partner.
When two leopards hunt, they often separate temporarily
to improve their chances to obtain a kill.

About six hours went by at our camera shelter in the bush. The heat became intense. Only a few antelopes passed by us. We went on waiting for something to film. Robert and Peter, the two Americans who were on the photo expedition with us, wanted to go back to camp. I was prepared to spend the night here. They thought I was crazy. I explained that I thought this area had something to offer my camera, and I didn't want to miss the opportunity. Peter and Robert decided to go back to camp. So with Mutero they set out for camp with the promise of returning the next day with food. Waiting in the same area for a long time usually proved worthwhile for filming.

SIGHTS AND SOUNDS OF AFRICA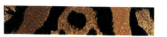

An hour later darkness fell. The night turned deep black. The monkeys chattered. Through the earphones of my tape recorder I listened to the sounds of the night and fell asleep. But the animals didn't fall asleep. Everything seemed to be awake and taking part in the nightly concert of the bush. I woke up repeatedly and stared into the gloom. Sometime during the night a big herd of buffalo or elephant sounded as if it were close by. The fear of being trampled made it difficult to sleep. I looked at my watch. It was four in the morning. At this point I could forget about sleep. The noise of the animals was incredibly loud. The first morning light on the horizon always thrilled and amazed me.

As I was setting up my camera I heard voices. It was Peter, Robert and Mutero. They slipped into the hideout. I wondered why they came back so early. Peter said they were eager to see if I was still alive. We decided to spend the day in the hideout in hopes of getting some good photos. We had just started breakfast when a warthog appeared.

About ten yards (9 meters) away it stopped dead, dropped to its knees, and started digging with its tusks. It brought out some roots and started to chew them. A slight noise brought it rapidly to its feet, then it quickly ran off. The next few hours went by with no sign of game. We took turns in sleeping and keeping watch. During the afternoon the scene suddenly changed within seconds. There was a grey wall of elephants on the far side of the waterhole. There must have been about two hundred of them. Leading them was a large bull. He first checked the area to see if it was clear. The only animal at the waterhole was a warthog and he was quickly chased away. More and more animals came streaming out of the bush and to the waterhole.

After drinking and splashing, two huge bull elephants seemed to be heading directly for us. "Careful," I gasped, and we all held our breaths in fear. I grabbed my rifle, while Peter pressed the camera button and Robert operated the tape recorder. Within a short time we were surrounded by elephants. They were trumpeting loudly. Panic gripped us. We were all in fear for our lives. Suddenly I remembered what an old tribesman had told me many years before. I took two sticks and beat them together, slowly at first then faster and louder. As the noise increased and grew faster the elephants began to move away. Within fifteen minutes there wasn't an elephant to be seen. They vanished into the bush. Everything was peaceful again.

Peter had filmed everything and Robert had kept the tape recorder running. We were so excited by this event that we decided to spend another night in the hideout in hopes of another showing. We ate our supper and tried to get some sleep.

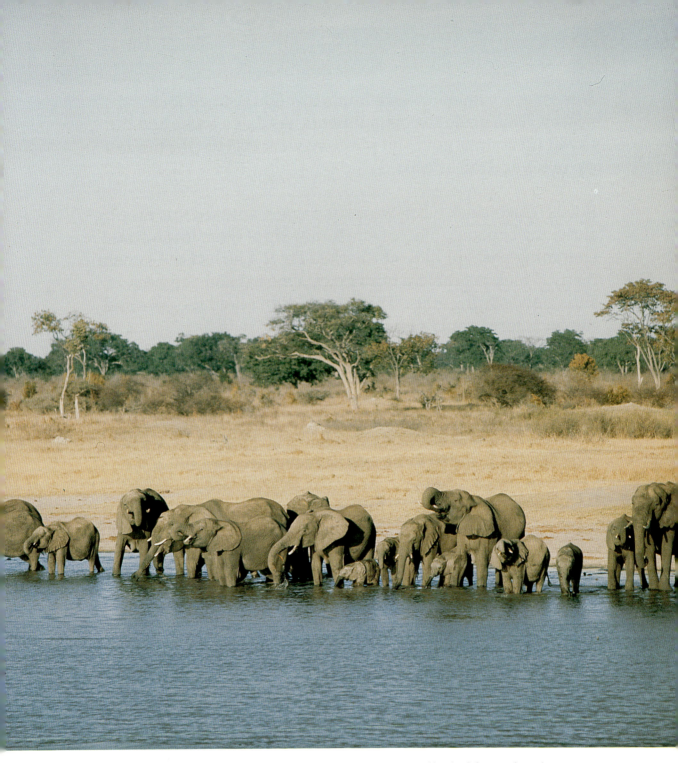

An extended family of elephants, usually led by a dominant "grandmother," moves everywhere together to exploit the resources of its huge home range in a controlled way.

Almost every animal which hunts by night seemed to be nearby. This made sleeping difficult. As dawn broke and the sky lit up orange, gold and pink, we were able to take our last sip of tea and fall asleep.

It was nine o'clock when we awoke again, aroused this time by shrieking baboons. There were hundreds of them leaping and chattering past our hideout. I asked Peter if he had the camera ready. I took the camera from Peter. One baboon had been sitting and staring at us. The baboon didn't hold the pose and ran off before I could film him.

Suddenly we saw a leopard slinking through the high grass. This was the reason the baboons were leaving us. A second leopard could be very close to us. We scanned the area for its possible companion. We spotted it in a mopani (mo-PAN-ee) tree. It was clear that these two were partners in a hunt.

We were aware that at any moment they might begin their stalking. A single baboon had remained in a nearby tree, not realizing the danger. With a quick spring, one leopard leapt into a tree next to the one in which the baboon sat. Then it crossed over to the baboon's tree. Horrified, the baboon fell out of the tree. It had hardly reached the ground when the second leopard took it by the neck. At that moment the first leopard jumped from the tree and tried to run off with the prey. But the killer leopard didn't want to share the meal. It growled and spat angrily at the other leopard. It took the prey and lodged it in the fork of a high tree, then returned to its partner as if nothing had happened. The two lay along side each other for three hours. They didn't move so much as a paw. By now it was very hot and the sun would soon be going down. We decided to spend one more night in the hideout.

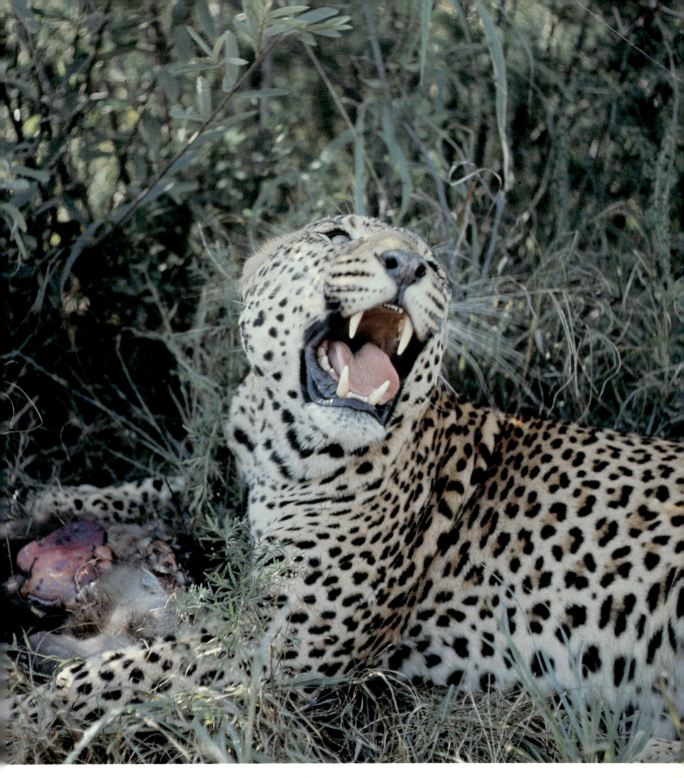

After it has first eaten, a leopard will often take the remains of large prey into a tree to keep it safe from scavengers.

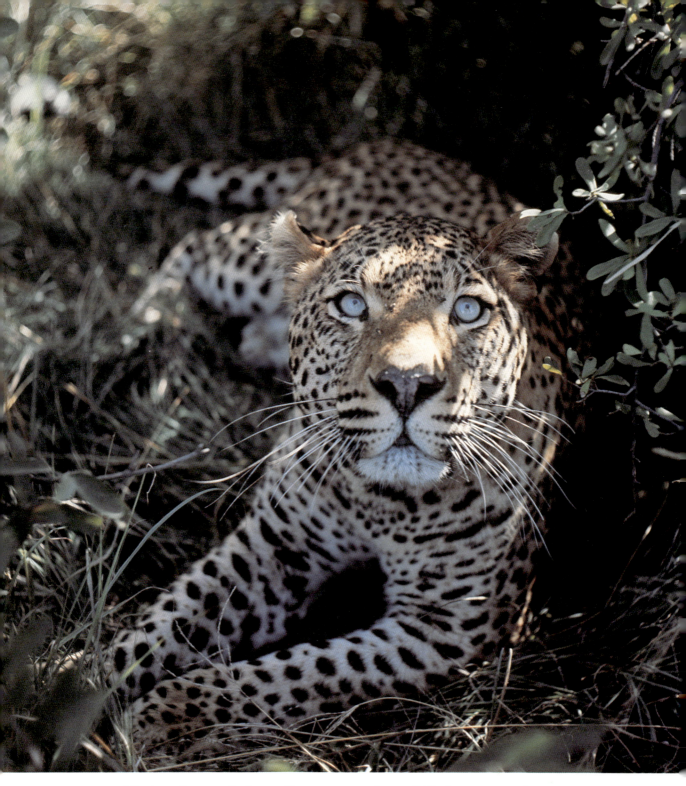

No two leopards have the same spots and their eyes are brown except when they reflect the blue sky.

Darkness came, and with it the noises of the baboons. They appeared to be sitting around the waterhole. They did not stop chattering all night. Many animals came close to us and left again. I was nervous about elephants and hippos, and I had also seen rhinos before in this area. If a rhino is startled it can become a dangerous and tricky enemy. Any of these thick-skinned creatures could have trampled us to death in our hide-out.

The night's sleep was terrible. We had to sleep crouching and half-standing. It was very hard on the back. It was unusually cold, and we were all freezing. Peter, Robert and Mutero decided to leave in the afternoon, but I was going to stay one more night. There were no animals to be seen at the moment. The heat was increasing, and all the animals were resting in the shade. Far and wide we couldn't see anything but dry grass and a couple of mopani trees.

Robert, Peter and Mutero left, promising to come back the next day. Suddenly, big herds of buffalo appeared on both sides of the waterhole. One herd on the far side was running towards the water, which is unusual. Another herd advanced more slowly, in the normal way. A third herd passed dangerously close to me.

I then filmed two bulls fighting. A single buffalo wandered off on its own along the waterside. It got a nasty shock when it encountered a crocodile. Next I heard the trumpeting of elephants. Shortly afterwards they broke out of the bush and rushed down to drink. Luckily there were none on my side of the waterhole. If so, I could have been trampled. I found myself thinking about elephants.

The living space for elephants is becoming smaller and smaller. It is almost impossible to make enough space available for their requirements. In the dry season elephants cover a distance of 19 to 25 miles (30 to 40 kilometers) a day. It is difficult for them to exist in areas without enough vegetation. They will eat everything. Several elephants will combine to push over and uproot large trees. The heavy, bony ridge at the base of their trunks is used for pushing. The tusks are used for levering and digging out.

THE AFRICAN ELEPHANT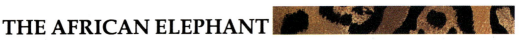

Elephants are skilled at finding underground water. They dig into the ground with their tusks. Depending on how hot it is, an elephant needs 90 to 135 quarts (85 to 127 liters) of water per day.

If you watch elephants at a waterhole, you can see that obedience is bred in these animals. The youngsters know that the elders come first. Elephants are delighted when the opportunity for a bath or a swim presents itself. They fill their trunks with water for drinking. They often take a shower by spraying the water over their own backs. Sometimes they duck under the surface, sticking their trunks out of the water so that they can breathe. It is amusing to watch elephants have a communal bath. In this game their togetherness shows up most of all. After its bath, the elephant sucks sand into its trunk and powders its whole body. Elephants have a great enjoyment of water. As they approach it, they give forth rumbles of pleasure that can be heard for several miles.

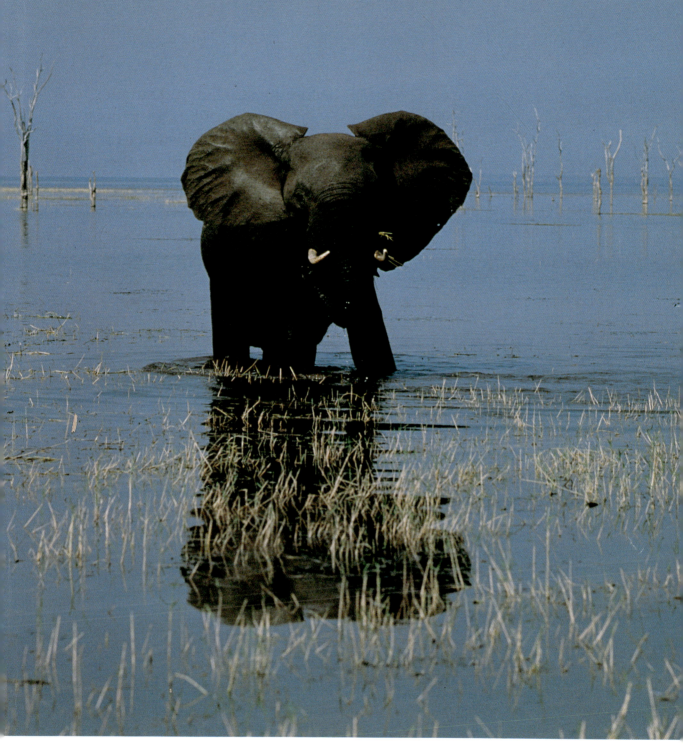

Untamed, fearless, independent, the African elephant has survived best in the parts of Africa remote from expanding populations of its only real enemy, mankind. Raised ears might indicate alarm - or merely that the animal is cooling itself.

Elephants have a total of 24 teeth. They use the front teeth the most, especially to strip bark from trees. The elephant eats for fifteen to twenty hours a day, so it only sleeps for three or four hours a day. The elephant loses its first teeth at the age of four or five. Once all its teeth have worn down and it cannot chew its food any longer, an elephant might die at forty or fifty years.

The elephant has little to fear in life except lack of food and water. Man is its only enemy. Because of man, all animals have been banished to live in smaller areas than they need to survive.

The elephant is a unique phenomenon in the animal world. Not only is it the biggest, the strongest and heaviest, its shape and behavior are completely different from other animals. The elephant has appendages to its vertical skull: large ears, a trunk and tusks.

The elephant's nose is extended into a trunk which has many uses apart from smelling, grasping and sucking. The trunk grabs leaves and twigs and feeds them into the mouth. Unlike any other animal, the elephant can use its trunk to feel out its surroundings. Thanks to its trunk it doesn't have to bend down to drink.

The ears are large and flat, and used for cooling. A standing elephant cools itself in the heat by moving the ears to and fro. The ear is full of fine veins which regulate the temperature of the whole body. The eyes are small and the elephant does not see very well. It is very graceful on its large feet. It moves so lightly that it is often seen before it is heard.

Its size and strength alone makes the elephant the true king of the animal kingdom. There are two kinds of elephants found in Africa. The larger of the two, the bush elephant, lives in southern Africa. Elephants prefer more densely wooded or bushy areas, which suit their feeding habits.

The average weight of the African elephant is six tons (5443 kilograms). The heaviest elephant ever found weighed 12 tons (10,886 kilograms). The longest tusks ever found were 10 feet (3.3 meters) and weighed 234 pounds (106 kilograms).

The elephants of southern Africa have long tails, sometimes reaching almost to the ground. The tail has thick wiry bristles at the end. The local people turn the bristles into rings and bracelets which are worn for good luck.

The adult elephants are dignified, quiet and restrained. The herds are rather noisy and the young bulls are high-spirited. They chase one another and other animals with a shrill squeal and loud, playful trumpeting. Half-grown bulls measure their strength by pushing against each other with the base of their trunks.

All ranges of trumpeting, from bass to soprano, can be heard from elephants going to the waterhole. The bulls travel on the outside of the herd. The cows and the young travel in the center, with small babies running almost under their mothers' stomachs.

The elephant's lordly status in the animal kingdom is evidenced by the way all others give way to them at the waterhole.

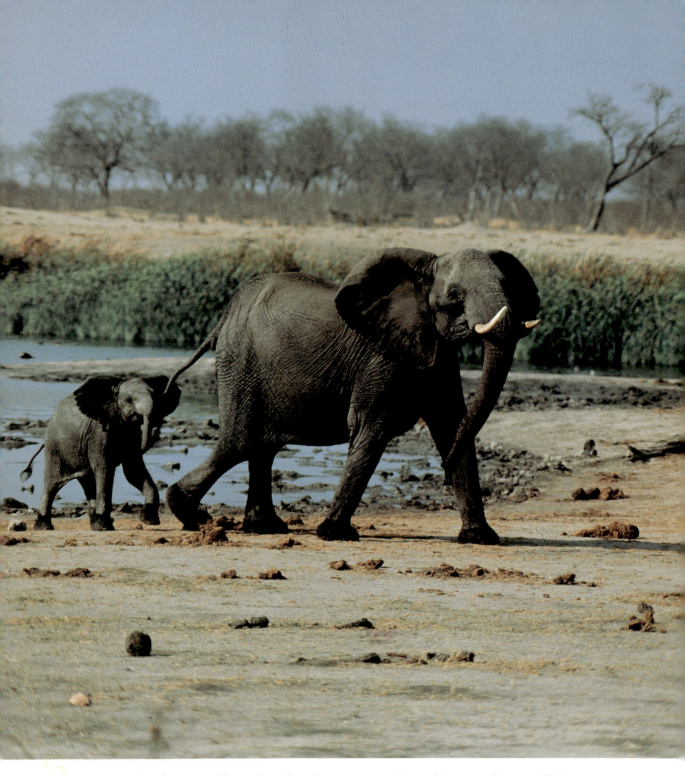

An elephant calf, under the close protection of its mother, will be weaned at two years old, but will not be fully grown until it is twenty-five. An elephant's normal life span is seventy years.

This seems only fair, since they are responsible for providing other animals with the watering facilities. I have seen them drive off lions from the waterhole to let the antelopes drink in safety. Often they trample crocodiles to death if they encounter them at a waterhole.

With their long legs, elephants move at a leisurely stroll of about 4 miles/hr (6 km/hr). They can stride up to 10 miles/hour (16 km/hr) when they are alarmed. When charging or fleeing in terror they can reach speeds of up to 25 miles/hr (40 km/hr).

Because of their size, elephants need large stretches of well-vegetated land and plenty of water. Their diets consist of leaves, shoots, reeds, bark, palm nuts, roots, seedpods and fruit.

A solid citizen, with strong family feelings, the elephant displays the confidence of superior intelligence. It dies more frequently from accident, old age and disease than hostile action from another animal. The herd protects the young and the sick. The worst danger the elephants face is a big brush fire. Brush fires move so fast and burn so fiercely that the elephants' thick skin can't even protect them.

If an elephant can't walk down a hill on its four feet, it will slide down the hill on its haunches. I saw this when I was filming in the Binga area. I was walking down a mountainside full of shrubs, gazing downward to look for footholds. When I glanced up, I saw 40 elephants sitting down on their haunches, sliding over the shrubs and stones on their backsides with their legs in the air.

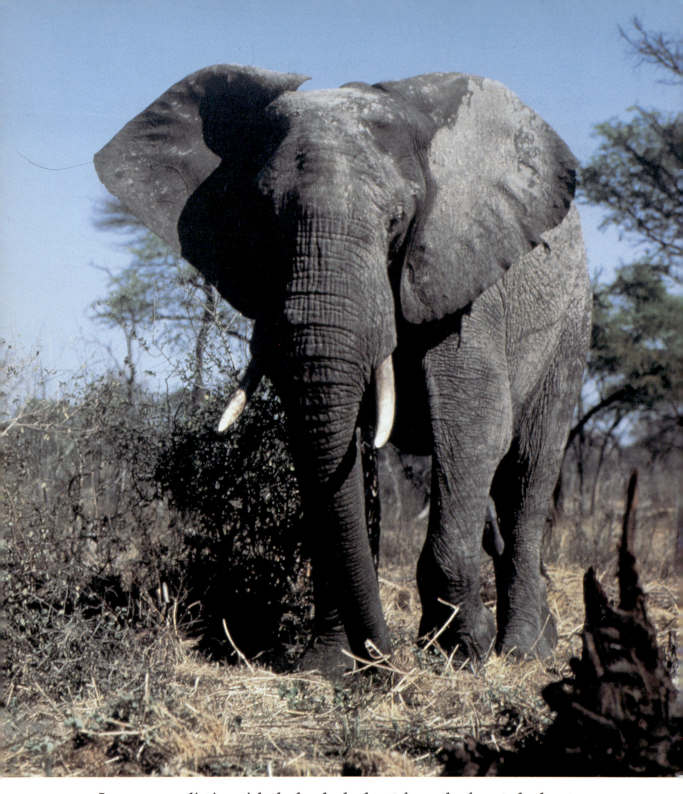

Larger ears distinguish the bush elephant from the forest elephant. There are many different types of elephants in Africa.

They were sliding as far as 300 feet (91 meters), squealing for joy. Some of them zig-zagged their way down, others forged straight ahead. They easily recovered their footing. This was one of the funniest scenes I had ever seen in the animal world.

Small elephants are protected by the whole herd, not just by the mother. I was once motoring down a narrow road with dense bush on either side when I encountered an elephant head-on in the middle of the road. It had its trunk raised. It was joined by a second and a third, which took up positions behind the first one. It was as if they were warning me. We waited patiently. Suddenly, a baby elephant, only a few days old, came out of the bush under another elephant's stomach and crossed the road. When it passed, the other elephants turned and followed.

Once Mutero and I were camping near the Savuti (Sah-VOO-tee) River. Almost each day small herds of elephants would play and swim in the river. One day on the opposite side of the river there was a large herd of buffalo. They smelled so bad that we had to move our camp. As we were moving we heard a loud thundering sound. We climbed a tree and saw what was coming. It was a huge herd of elephant pushing their way through the buffalo. It was fascinating to watch, especially how the buffalo allowed the elephants to push their way through. Even the buffalo leader looked for another path to take. More and more elephants pushed their way to the river. As they got closer to the water they began to run faster and faster. When they reached the river, the elephants plunged into the water. It turned different colors from the dust on their backs.

I had become so interested in this wonderful sight that I had not noticed that Mutero had climbed down from the tree. He soon told me to climb down as well. By that time the elephants had reached our side of the river and were climbing the bank. We quickly slipped away, out of the dust, and were glad to be safe.

ANIMALS OF THE OKAVANGO DELTA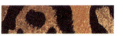

On another occasion, it was October, and as usual it was very hot. We were resting on an island west of the Okavango (Oh-kah-VON-go). A few ivory palm trees cast some shade. In the heat of the afternoon sun, I fell asleep. Suddenly one of my assistance woke me. I sat up, still half asleep and looked across at the water. I saw something moving in the distance. At first, I thought it was a boat. Then I realized it was part of an elephant's head. The body was not visible at all. I could only see the trunk. It was moving like a snorkel through the water. I didn't know how deep the water was at that spot or whether the elephant was walking or swimming. From its movements it looked more as if it were swimming. Then we saw that it was not alone. Several elephants followed the leader from one island to another. They were all completely submerged with only their trunks sticking out of the water. As they made their way out of the water, we saw that there were older and younger elephants of different sizes. It must have been impossible for the younger ones to touch the bottom. I came to the conclusion that they had to be swimming, despite the belief that elephants can't swim.

The morning after Mutero and I had seen the elephants and buffalo herd together, the whole area seemed dead. Around midday, hippos appeared and eventually came out of the water on the opposite bank.

They were lying peacefully in the sun. But it didn't last. We soon heard elephants trumpeting. This time it was a smaller herd, all bulls, which appeared out of the bushes and made their way to the water. They were not happy to have their path to the water being blocked by the hippos. The leader of the hippos refused to move. So one of the biggest elephants advanced on the hippo and pushed it. The two ton hippo lost its balance and tumbled into the water. The hippo was furious, and kept surfacing and spraying the elephant in protest. But it always kept its distance from the elephant. As the elephants entered the water the hippos disappeared under the water, as if they had never been there at all.

During the night we were suddenly awakened. Elephants were all around us. They got tangled up in our tent. The whole thing collapsed. Fortunately it was the tent which had been prepared for our guests from the United States, so it was empty. I asked Mutero to put as much wood on the fire as possible. This kept the elephants away. Soon they made off into the darkness, leaving us very tired, but wakeful with the excitement. I lay awake for a long time, asking myself, who were the intruders, us or them?

When I was living in camp alone with Joseph and his wife, I was often visited by wild animals which were curious without being dangerous. Perhaps they had accepted me in their surroundings. Among the most frequent visitors were elephants. There was one young elephant which visited me several mornings. He would run and look around the camp for things to eat. One day I decided to try and film him in action. I set the camera on automatic and Joseph and I went about our normal tasks. While both of us had our backs turned, the elephant wandered into the tent.

Completely unaware of its presence, I went on with my break-fast. Imagine my surprise when the elephant appeared out of the tent and draped its trunk over my shoulder. I fed it what was left on my plate. That seemed to satisfy it. Then I followed it to locate the rest of the herd.

Darkness fell and I was beginning to nod off in my hideout. I regained my alertness as the night noises started up. Some of them were peaceful and some were aggressive. After awhile I fell asleep. It was still dark, however, when I was shocked awake by the shelter collapsing on me. I was half asleep, and just for a moment I couldn't grasp the situation. If I had been attacked by an animal I wouldn't have realized it in my daze. After the first shock, I grabbed my rifle and fired a shot into the air. I then raised myself from the debris. There were dark shadows all around me. It was a herd of buffalo. I was in the middle. There were quite a few big bulls around me. I sat very still and waited for them to go away. Then the sun rose, and one by one the buffalo began to go about their business.

I looked for all the equipment and then packed the camera away carefully. At the same time I found a can of condensed milk. I swallowed the entire contents. After an hour, one bull was still directly behind me. Finally, it moved off, followed by the rest of the buffalo in the area. I breathed a sigh of relief and moved out of the remains of my shelter, always keeping an eye on the buffalo. Suddenly it occurred to me that lions might be near.

Then I saw something peeping out of a hole in the tree. It was a dwarf mongoose. Its head was popping in and out. I got my camera to film the mongoose, but nothing happened.

I started to feel drowsy again, forcing myself to keep my eyes open. After what seemed like forever, the mongoose appeared again. It stuck its head out of the tree, then came out with its long tail waving like a flag. In a split second it was out of sight again, but I had captured it on film.

THE AFRICAN MONGOOSE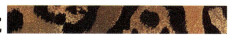

Mongooses are among the most popular of African small game. The smallest is the dwarf or pygmy mongoose. It is a small grayish-brown animal with a body of 8 inches (20 centimeters) and a tail of 5 inches (12.7 centimeters). They are found in bushy country where they move in small troops.

Depending on the species, mongooses look as if they belong to the cat family. A person can easily tell the different types of mongoose. They have body lengths ranging from 8 to 26 inches (20 to 66 centimeters), the tail often being as long as the body.

On many occasions I have watched banded mongooses. Their body is about 10 inches (25 centimeters) long. They have dark stripes over the back of their grey coat. This animal has a pink snout and feet. The tail, which is 5 inches (12.7 centimeters) long, is darker than the body and has a blackish tip. The soles of their feet are naked to the heel. The upper lip is divided. They are extremely active little animals, chattering to each other all the time. When cross they growl harshly. They have no fixed home. They move from burrow to burrow, sometimes nesting in trees. They are very curious animals.

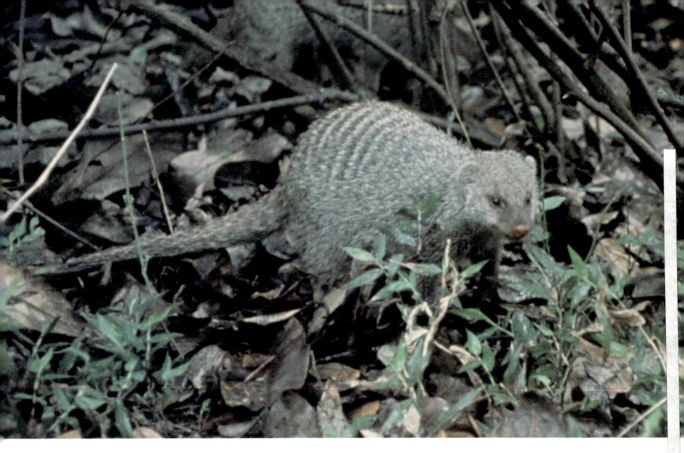

The African banded mongoose.

Mongooses feed on insects, grubs, small rodents, eggs, young birds, and small reptiles. Snake-killing is their speciality. Snakes are usually attacked by two mongooses with impressive footwork and strategy.

Banded mongooses often used to visit my camp and steal eggs. They hunt all types of eggs: birds', snakes', or fowls' eggs. To open the eggs, they have worked out a very clever trick. They take the egg in their front paws and sling it backwards through their hind legs to shatter it on a stone or log.

Over the years that I have studied wild animals, I have come to understand them more and more. I am always happy when they visit my camp. When possible, I even encourage them to do so.

THE ZEBRA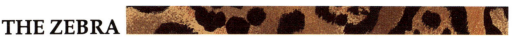

When wandering in the bush, I always carry some food with me in case I am stranded. On one of my walks, I came across a herd of zebra. A young zebra was standing apart from the herd. I decided to try and make friends with it. I crept up slowly towards it, holding out some candy I had in my pocket. The zebra smelled it, but showed no further interest. I threw the candy on the ground because it had become sticky. To my surprise, I saw the zebra lower its head to eat the candy. I offered it more candy and eventually it ate from my hands. We spent the afternoon together and I was lucky enough to witness a zebra close up.

Zebra have a steadier personality than the wildebeest. The family units in which they live promote stability. Zebra families usually consist of a stallion, several mares and their foals.

Adults stay with their family for life but stallions leave on their own to join other bachelors. Even when a family joins another family to form a larger herd, each family keeps its identity. The stripe pattern of each zebra is as distinctive as a human finger-print.

With their rich and strongly-marked stripes, zebras are the most decorative of the African animals. The most common zebra in southern Africa is Burchell's zebra. Burchell's is more fully striped than zebra found in other parts of Africa. Their build is like a horse or pony. The shoulder height is 54 inches (137 centimeters) and they weigh 661 pounds (300 kilograms). For some reason zebra always seem to be plump.

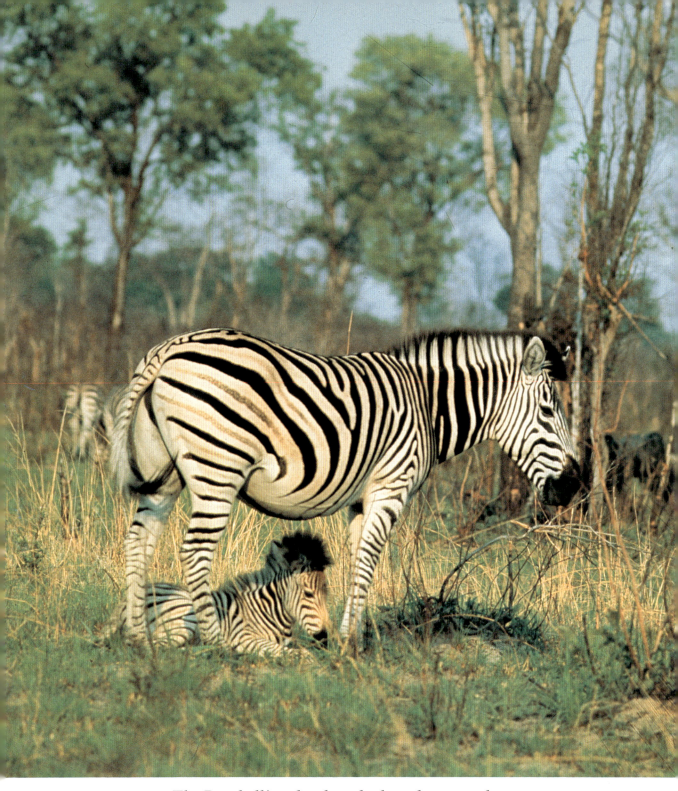

*The Burchell's zebra has shadows between the
dark stripes that also continue under the belly.*

Zebra move in troops of about twenty, increasing to hundreds when searching for water. They often associate with antelopes such as wildebeest, kudu, impala, nyala, and sometimes even with buffalo herds. These animals seem to depend on the zebra to be their lookout and to warn them if danger is near.

Zebra are restless and noisy, with a cry like a barking whinny. It is soothing to hear zebra braying at night. Their wild and haunting calls fill the space between the stars and the Earth. Zebra eat only grass, and are found on the open plains.

Their main enemy is the lion. Their means of self-defense is kicking and biting. The males fight each other savagely during the mating season and at the waterholes. Their search for water takes them far and wide.

I once made an interesting discovery when I was in the bush all alone, trying to record bird sounds. With much patience I was able to entice a young zebra to stay by me for hours. I recorded its braying and other sounds of the wilderness.

Burchell's zebra is known for its shadows between the dark stripes. It also has stripes under the belly. This is the main difference between the Burchell's and the Hartmann's zebra. There are only a few specimen of the Hartmann's zebra left in the world. They are mostly found in African game reserves but even there they are slowly dying out. They are very shy, and are seldom seen outside the game reserves. Those that still exist know how to avoid human beings. Wherever possible, the few remaining Hartmann's zebra are being moved to game reserves to prevent extinction.

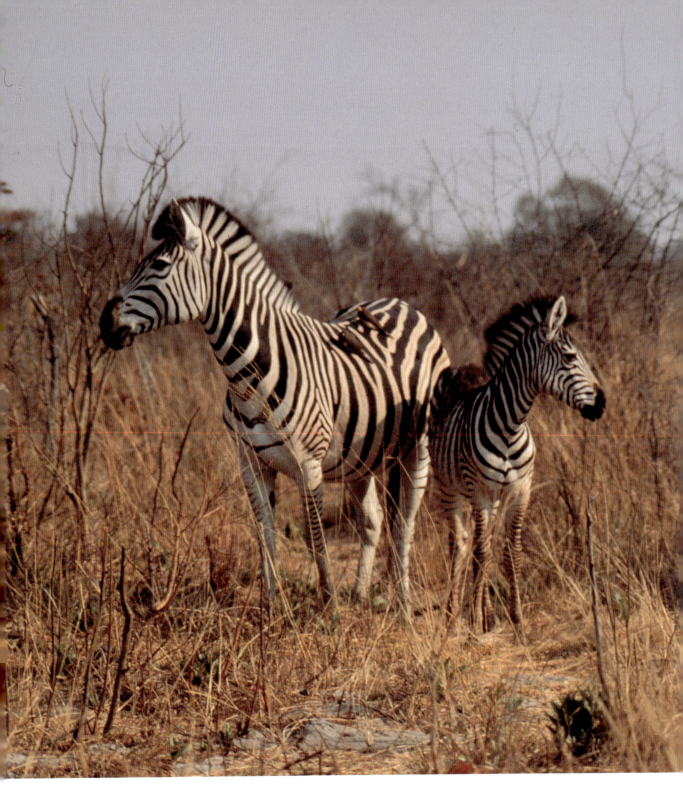

Zebra foals always stay close to their mothers. The zebra foal tends to stand out in the group, especially on the open plain.

I experienced their shyness myself when I once saw a group of eight. It was interesting to see that the leader of the group was a female. It was easy to recognize them as Hartmann's zebra: their stripes are wider than those of Burchell's zebra, and the belly is white with no stripes at all. They are more alert than the other types of zebra. They are very hard to approach. They measure about 50 inches (127 centimeters) at the shoulder.

THE NYALA

Another animal which was thought at one time to be almost extinct is the nyala (nee-AH-la). It was once considered one of the rarest antelopes in southern Africa. However, it is more prominent than previously believed. The nyala is one of the most secretive antelopes. It only comes out at night to feed.

The nyala male stands about 42 inches (106 centimeters) at the shoulder and is brown in color. It has a few white stripes down its side. On the neck a black mane goes back to the shoulders. The nose is marked by a white "V" between the eyes. The twisted, yellow-tipped horns are big. They are about 24 inches (61 centimeters) in length. The tail is long and bushy, black above and white underneath.

The females are usually hornless. They have shorter tails than the males. They are bright chestnut-red in color. There is no "V" on the face. I have on one occasion seen a female with horns, but this is very rare. I was lucky enough to film the animal as it hid behind some bushes.

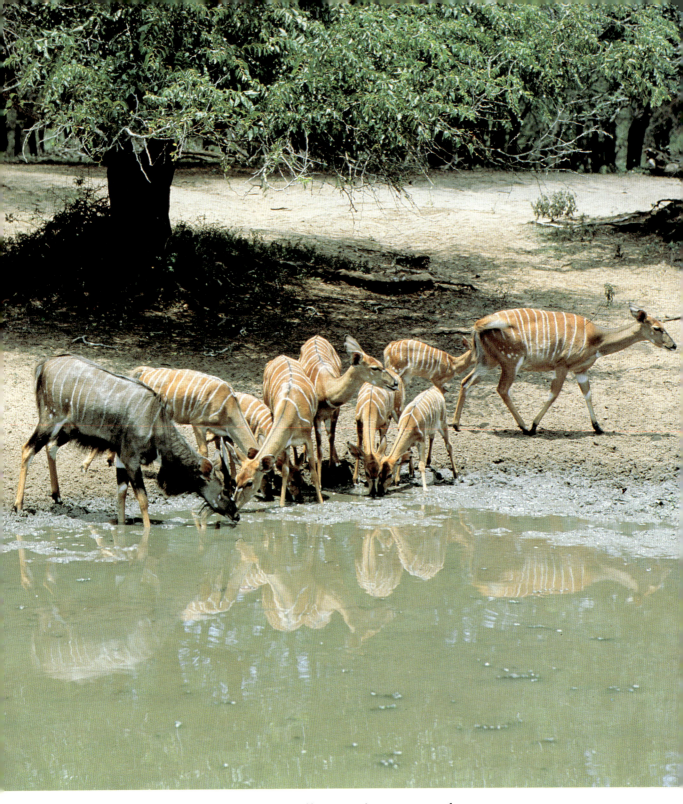

Nyalas are usually seen in groups of two or three females and a few males.

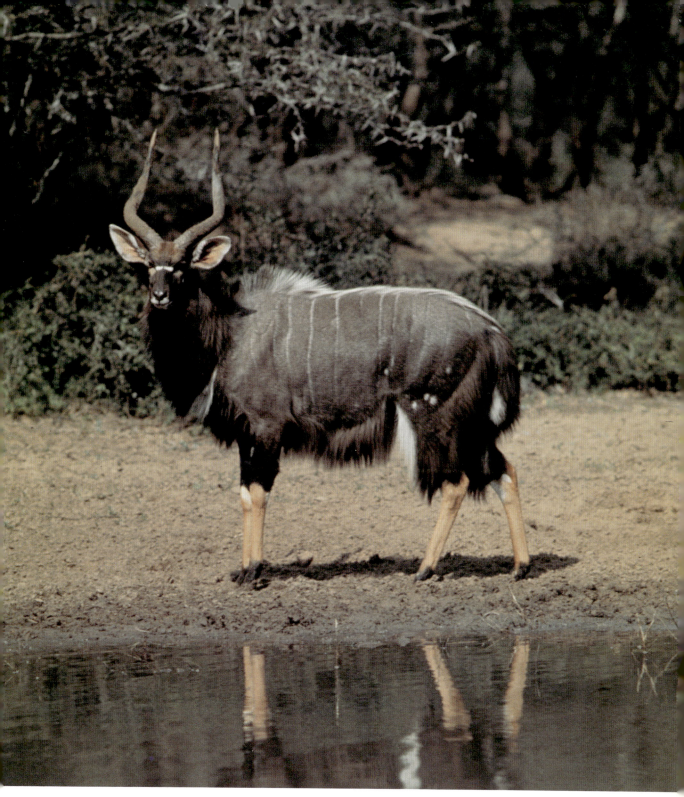

The nyala has a black mane that goes as far as the shoulders, with a white "V" between the eyes.

Nyala are seen in small groups. When running they turn up their tails like most antelopes do.

I decided to go on waiting for more shots of leopards. I went back to the ruins of my hideout. I was completely exhausted and couldn't keep myself from falling asleep. I'm not sure what woke me up. I heard a muffled growl, and saw a leopard barely 23 feet (7 meters) away from me. It was looking at me. I picked up my rifle very quickly. I had it under my arm as the leopard took a few slow steps closer to me. The distance between us now was only 13 feet (4 meters). I risked taking out my camera, never taking my eyes off the leopard. I tried to get the correct focus and press the button. But the leopard had other ideas. It turned away from me and made its way to a dead baboon that was hanging in the fork of a tree. It was difficult keeping up with it. The leopard would not like me following it. My rifle was at the ready. I focused my camera when the leopard jumped into the tree and crept toward its prey for a snack. I was lucky to have filmed this whole scene. The leopard then climbed out of the tree and vanished into the bush.

The long hard wait had really been worth it. Happily I returned to the hideout. I put all my things together and went back to the camp. I had the once-in-a-lifetime luck to film leopards hunting and returning to their prey. These animals only appear at night, which makes filming impossible. After walking a few hundred feet towards the camp, Mutero rushed out to meet me. He took my load from me and asked me what I had seen. But I was too exhausted to talk.

I needed all my energy to return to camp. For several days I had not washed and my skin felt almost dried out. I began to doubt whether I would make it back to camp. The last few miles seemed to last forever. When I arrived in camp, Peter came towards me and welcomed me. He looked at me and asked how I felt, but I just shook my head. I found my bed and fell into a deep sleep. The next morning Mutero woke me with a cup of tea. I swallowed that and fell asleep again. Towards midday I woke up again, feeling rested. I also felt very hungry. I ate a huge breakfast, probably the biggest I have ever eaten in my life. Then I began to tell them what had happened...

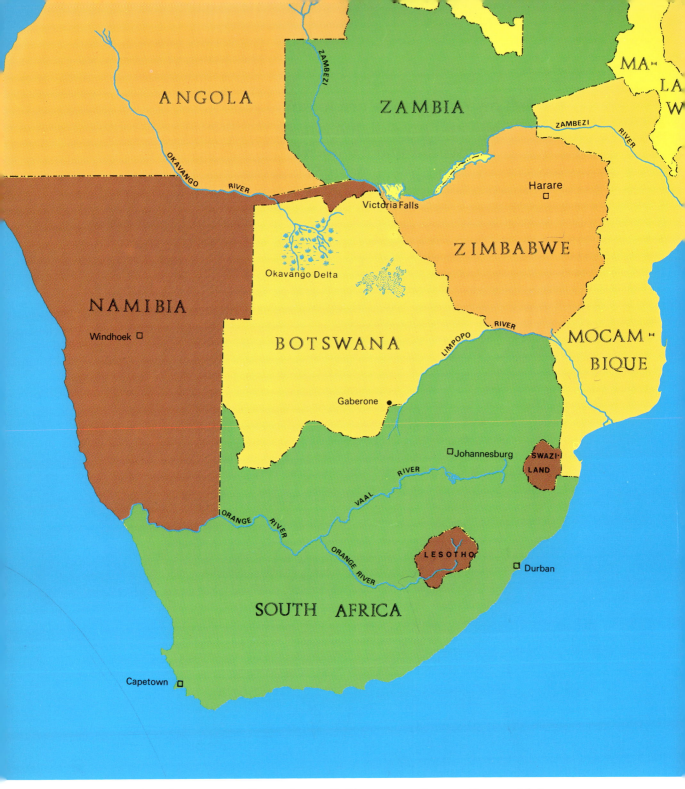

ANGOLA

ZAMBIA

ZAMBEZI

ZAMBEZI RIVER

MALAW

OKAVANGO RIVER

Harare

Victoria Falls

ZIMBABWE

Okavango Delta

NAMIBIA

Windhoek

BOTSWANA

MOCAM-BIQUE

LIMPOPO RIVER

Gaberone

Johannesburg

SWAZI-LAND

RIVER

VAAL

ORANGE RIVER

ORANGE RIVER

LESOTHO

Durban

SOUTH AFRICA

Capetown

Our journey took us through Botswana in southern Africa.
We travelled through the Kalahari Desert into the Okavango Delta.

GLOSSARY

Africa - a continent (large body of land) south of the Mediterranean Sea between the Atlantic and Indian Ocean.

Antelope - a swift-running animal resembling a deer, found especially in Africa.

Baboon - a large African monkey.

Binga - an area in the Okavango delta of southern Africa.

Buffalo - a kind of ox found in Asia and southern Africa.

Bush - wild, remote, uncultivated land.

Bushman - a member of an aboriginal tribe of southern Africa.

Crocodile - a large reptile with thick skin, a long tail, and huge jaws.

Cub - the young of certain animals such as, fox, bear, lion.

Elephant - a very large land animal with a trunk and long curved ivory tusks.

Expedition - a journey for a particular purpose.

Herd - a number of animals feeding or staying together.

Hippopotamus - a large African river animal with tusks, short legs, and thick skin.

Ivory Palm Tree - western African trees with large leaves.

Leopard - a large African and Asian flesh-eating animal of the cat family.

Lion - a large, powerful African and Asian flesh-eating animal of the cat family.

Mongoose - a small weasel-like animal that kills snakes.

Mopani Tree - a tree found in the desert regions of southern Africa.

Nyala - an antelope-like animal.

Okavango Delta - an area of the country of Botswana which is plentiful in water and wildlife.

Prey - an animal that is hunted or killed by another for food.

Reedbuck - an average size antelope.

Reptiles - cold-blooded animals with a backbone, short legs or no legs; lizard.

Rhinoceros - a large thick-skinned African animal possessing a horn on its nose.

Rodent - an animal with strong front teeth used for gnawing things; rat, squirrel.

Savuti Channel - a narrow waterway of the Savuti River in Botswana, Africa.

Tusk - one of a pair of long pointed teeth that project outside the mouth in certain animals.

Warthog - a kind of African pig with two large tusks and warts on its face.

Wildebeest - an ox-like animal or gnu.

Zebra - an African animal of the horse family, covered with black and white stripes.

Index